CBD HEMP OIL

A Natural Alternative for Disease Treatment and Pain Relief

Christopher Knowles

Table of Contents

Cannabidiol Oil

When someone mentions the word marijuana a ton of different passionate and vocal opinions begin to surface. Marijuana has been a plant of controversy for decades. This plant was once given the opportunity to provide its benefits legally in the United States in the 1940's; however, when policymakers determined the high abuse potential related with this plant, they decided it was too good for the American people, and band it from the United States. Thus, making marijuana illegal.

Now we all know, that while the political leaders may have deemed marijuana illegal, it did not diminish the use of this plant by millions of individuals for recreational use, on a daily basis. People decided to incorporate marijuana into their lifestyles for a variety of reasons. Some of those reasons include the frivolous and irresponsible reason, "to get high." Other more responsible reasons include: to treat nausea from chemotherapy, to treat seizures or other neurologic diseases, to increase appetite in cancer or AIDS patients, and other medical reasons.

Marijuana's medical benefits have been controversial to say the least; however, as we start to cross into the land of tolerability, more and more research is being conducted to determine just how much of an impact this plant will have on different medical conditions. There are over 24 states that have legalized the medical use of marijuana and its components. Let's take a look at one of these components and determine the benefits surrounding its use.

What is Cannabidiol Oil?

The Cannabis plant, is made up of many components. The two main components that are showing promising results regarding the research in which is being conducted include: THC and Cannabidiol. Cannabidiol is the non-psychoactive ingredient. Cannabidiol is the component that can be extracted from the different areas of the plant including both the marijuana portion and the hemp portion. Therefore, there is definitely some controversy on the legal side of things when determining which portion of the plant can be consumed. Whether, the Cannabidiol is received from the marijuana or hemp, it offers great possibilities for addressing symptoms associated with debilitating and devastating health conditions.

Cannabis is the actual plant and most scientists claim that the active ingredient, THC as the component that results in the "high" that drug abusers seek. Because marijuana is a plant and not made up of just one ingredient; there are other active ingredients that offer benefits without causing these the classic high seen with THC.

One of these active ingredients that is being researched across many medical spectrums is Cannabidiol Oil (CBD). CBD is an active ingredient found in the marijuana plant, that is offering promising results in treating rare medical conditions. CBD is also offering promising results in treating those medical conditions in which traditional therapies have failed.

Those medical conditions that CDB has offered benefits include: seizures, central nervous system disorders, peripheral nervous system disorders, anxiety, cancer, and other neurodegenerative disorders. These medical conditions have reeked havoc on the patients that have been diagnosed with these diseases; and so after trying traditional Western medicine with no sustainable outcomes, they have decided to explore other avenues that may provide them with some sort of relief. Because of the sense of vulnerability and defeat, these patients seeking alternative therapies are willing to try something that is controversial and still in its beginning stages of research, and that therapy is Cannabidiol Oil.

Cannabidiol Oil has a low level of psychoactive properties as compared to THC. The result is an ingredient that does not create "the high" effects that are normally observed with the consumption of THC. Cannabidiol Oil, while still in the beginning stages of research, is showing promising benefits when treating symptoms associated with many neurodegenerative disorders. Some disorders that Cannabidiol Oil is showing benefits in managing include: arthritis, diabetes, pain, anxiety, mental health disorders, epilepsy, and cancer. In the subcategory of mental health disorders, there are: depression, post-traumatic stress disorder, schizophrenia, and others.

These are only a short list of the neurological diseases and other miscellaneous diseases and symptoms that CBD Oil may have the potential to offer benefits. Now that we have established how specific components of marijuana can in fact offer potentially beneficial results in the healthcare world; let's begin by analyzing and making our own decision about this specific component: Cannabidiol Oil.

How is it Obtained?

When an individual is using CBD for medical therapeutic reasons, the goal is to extract as much pure CBD as possible to create the oil. Therefore, in order to receive the most pure content, we can extract this oil from the hemp portion of the plant. The hemp portion of the plant contains high levels of CBD and little to no levels of THC, the psychoactive ingredient of marijuana. CBD can be extracted from the marijuana flower portion as well, but there is a high concentration of THC levels in that part of the plant and so to separate the two components can result in a less pure form.

There are many different ways to actually perform extraction of CBD. The safety of extraction can vary and so it is imperative to make sure that a professional is the one that performs the extraction.

What is the United States Legal Status?

With all of the laws and regulations both federal and state-by-state, there can be some contradictory and confusing issues regarding what is legal and what is deemed illegal. One statement that to this day is still true is that marijuana and its components gathered from it are illegal as it is declared by Federal Law.

Since Cannabidiol Oil is a component of marijuana, then if this oil is extracted from the marijuana flower, it is considered illegal by Federal standards. However, this is not where this story ends. Because states have the flexibility to create their own legislation to a certain degree, there are states that have declared marijuana to be legal not only for medical purposes but also for recreational use. In those states that allow the legal use of marijuana, then in turn Cannabidiol Oil is also legal since it is obtained from the cannabis plant.

You may be thinking, well I don't live in one of the states that has become so progressive and has passed the law that states marijuana is legal for medical and recreational uses? But don't worry, I have the answer! One amazing fact about Cannabidiol Oil is that it not only comes from the marijuana flower, it is also a component of hemp. Yes, you heard me correctly. CBD Oil can be extracted from the hemp portion of the cannabis plant. This is an amazing breakthrough. Because of the important medical benefits this oil is proving to offer, many individuals have been seeking a way to get their hands on this product. However, many are discouraged because they find out it comes from marijuana and they know that it is illegal federally as well as where they live.

The best news I can provide is that Cannabidiol Oil is also extracted from hemp. Because hemp is deemed legal at all levels both federally and state-to-state, this means that any CBD Oil extracted from hemp can be legally purchased. Many different supplemental products that are being sold in nutrition and vitamin shops market these products to offer the benefits that so many people have been hoping for. Many researchers and scientists are looking to determine if these claims associated with CBD Oil are true. If they are, this oil can offer relief to those who were suffering from these diseases and felt like they had reached their end.

So now that we have laid out how Cannabidiol Oil can be obtained let's have a brief re-cap so that we can make sure the specific take home messages have been received. Basically, Cannabidiol Oil can be extracted from two portions of the Cannabis plant. CBD Oil can be extracted from marijuana and also extracted from the hemp portion of the plant. Because there is so much controversy across the United States about what is federally considered legal, and what is considered state-to-state legal, we have decided to separate the two types of CBD Oil based on the method in which they have been extracted.

First of all, CBD Oil obtained from Hemp is completely legal across all the states in the United States. CBD Oil extracted from hemp is considered a supplement and is sold in health food stores. Because there is not any significant levels of THC in this type of oil, it is considered to not offer any psychoactive characteristics and thus is not illegal. The other type of CBD Oil is extracted from the marijuana plant, and this oil is has high content of THC and has high content of CBD Oil; therefore, it is federally illegal.

As we have discussed, over the past few years in the United States, we have noticed that there are many states that have determined that not only medical marijuana is acceptable, but also the use of marijuana for recreational purposes has also become legal. In those states that have passed these laws, CBD Oil extracted from marijuana is legal according to the state laws, but is still federally illegal. One thing that is not so controversial and confusing, is that CBD offers a variety of benefits that range from pain relief to symptom relief of neurodegenerative diseases.

What are the effects of CBD Oil?

Most sources seem to agree that CBD Oil is probably safe. However, as with any supplement or medicine it is important to contact your healthcare provider concerning any specific addition to your healthcare treatment plan. All supplements and over-the-counter medications should be discussed with your doctor so that it can be determined there are no interactions that could result in adverse effects.

Side effects listed by WebMD, associated with Cannabidiol include: dry mouth, decrease in blood pressure, dizziness or lightheadedness, and drowsiness. Other side effects include the increased potential for Cannabidiol to interact with other drugs. Because of its specific type of metabolism, the consumption of this supplement may result in synergistic effects with some medications increasing their potency. Therefore, while Cannabidiol has been labeled as safe, anytime a patient is on more than one medication, supplement, or even over-the-counter medication there is a very high chance that interactions will occur.

As with every supplement or medicine it is imperative to exert extreme caution if a woman is currently pregnant, or intends to become pregnant. At this time there is not enough research to determine whether or not taking Cannabidiol is safe either during pregnancy or while breastfeeding. It is recommended that with any medication or supplement, that if there is not enough evidence to determine if Cannabidiol may result in harm to the fetus, or baby during breastfeeding, to avoid taking this supplement. The best option is to focus on the side of caution in these instances.

As we have stated earlier, there are two different ways in which to extract this Cannabidiol Oil, and depending on which portion of the cannabis plant this CBD Oil is extracted from, there can be different side effects that become evident. For example, if the CBD Oil is extracted from the marijuana flower component, it is extracted with some levels of THC. As we all know, THC is considered the psychoactive portion of marijuana. The THC is what results in an individual becoming "high" as a result of ingesting or smoking marijuana. So, it is understandable to come to the assumption that if CBD Oil is extracted from marijuana and some THC is also present; then other symptoms and side effects could potentially occur. However, those side effects would be as a result of ingesting the component THC, and not caused by the consumption of CBD Oil. So, we still consider the side effects of CBD Oil to be minimal and variable based on the individual and the types of medication interactions that may be present.

What Diseases is it believed to treat?

During the past several years medical marijuana and marijuana use for recreational purposes has been all over the news. Policymakers on a daily basis are providing support and then others are providing road blocks. Every Politician has a different stance on whether or not marijuana has any place in the medical field. One thing that policymakers cannot deny is that while they are trying to determine whether or not it has a potential to be medically beneficial, the scientists and physicians researching these areas have already concluded that there is significant reason to believe that there are benefits to be received from incorporating medical marijuana and its components into the healthcare of their patients. Scientists and physicians are also currently conducting research on the benefits of Cannabidiol Oil for treatment of many different symptoms and diseases.

Those symptoms range from chronic pain and chronic fatigue, to diseases such as Parkinson's disease, Alzheimer's or Dementia, Multiple Sclerosis, and Epilepsy. These neurodegenerative diseases affect collectively millions of people per year. These individuals are suffering from these diseases and are asking for research to show some type of promising results so that they can have hope of alleviating some of these symptoms, or even provide cures for specific diseases. There is great opportunity here to continue research and determine the scientific evidence-based information that will provide promising results on such a topic.

One online website that offers information about Cannabidiol is titled, Leaf Science. This website takes a look at some of the symptoms that CBD has offered specific benefits. Some of those properties that Cannabidiol Oil exhibits include the following: antiemetic, anticonvulsant, antipsychotic, anti-inflammatory, anti-oxidant, anti-tumor/anti-cancer, and anxiolytic/anti-depressant. This information was received from the Leaf Science website.

Those medical terms may seem overwhelming, but don't let that stand in your way of understanding how simple their interpretation can be. First of all, antiemetic refers to diminishing nausea and vomiting and research suggests that CBD oil can offer anti-nausea these effects.

Anticonvulsant effects associated with CBD Oil are one of the major areas that is being researched. The shear definition of Epilepsy is a seizure in which there is no known cause. Because there is not an underlying cause that can be treated, these individuals who suffer from seizures live in fear of when the next seizure will occur. It severely limits their ability to have a normal quality of life. These individual who suffer from Epilepsy as well as other seizure disorders are normally on anticonvulsant medications, and one beneficial effect of CBD Oil is that it offers additional anti seizure benefits.

Another important property of CBD is that it helps to provide antipsychotic benefits. Through research, scientists are beginning to understand how CBD Oil can actually offer benefits to those individuals who suffer from diseases such as Bipolar. A variety of

11

mental health populations have noticed a tremendous difference when CBD was incorporated into their lifestyle. CBD has also been showing promising results when exhibiting anti-anxiety and anti-depressive effects. Anxiety and Depression are two major diagnoses that plague our society more than ever. CBD Oil is showing promising results that will address these symptoms and disorders that impact so many in our society today.

CBD Oil can also act as an anti-inflammatory. This can be beneficial to those individuals who suffer from autoimmune diseases in which their own bodies are causing an increase in inflammation resulting in detrimental effects. Some outstanding research is even claiming that CBD Oil is offering promising results in anti-tumor and anti-cancer properties. This basically means that there is some research that is suggesting CBD Oil can cure cancer. While this claim may be far fetched, and there definitely needs to be more evidence based medicine to make this scientific claim, if it is proven to be true it would be a huge scientific breakthrough that would be an amazing discovery. Finally, antioxidant is another property that CBD Oil has, and thus helps to address the symptoms associated with neurodegenerative diseases.

As a patient, or a consumer, if you are looking through this information trying to determine which claims are true and which claims need to be researched more it is imperative to follow up on the research that has been conducted, and continues to be conducted, on the specific areas of interest. One source that offers more scientific, evidence-based medicine results concerning Cannabidiol is WebMD.

One medical condition that there has been significant evidence to prove that Cannabidiol does offer significant benefits is in those patients who suffer from Multiple Sclerosis. Multiple Sclerosis is defined by Medscape as, "an immune-mediated inflammatory disease that attacks myelinated axons in the central nervous system, destroying the myelin and the axon in a variable degrees and producing significant physical disability within 20-25 years in more than 30% of patients."

Say what? So, basically Multiple Sclerosis is a disease that affects the central nervous system. The central nervous system is classified as the brain and the spinal cord. It is an inflammatory disease that actually takes off the protective covering that the nerves have. That protective covering that allows for the transmittance of signals is called myelin. When that protective covering is damaged and deteriorated, then symptoms begin to occur, and physical disabilities appear. Multiple Sclerosis is a progressive disease that causes patients a lot of physical pain. WebMD explains that Cannabidiol has been proven to offer significant benefits.

The treatment for Multiple Sclerosis is actually a nasal spray that is a prescription that patients receive from their physician. The prescription is called Sativex. Sativex is a nasal spray that actually contains both THC and Cannabidiol. The reason this is prescribed to patients is to provide pain relief, provide relief of muscle tightness, and urinary frequency. This treatment method has been observed in many other countries as a standard in which many individuals with Multiple Sclerosis have benefited. This treatment is currently in the clinical trial phase in the United States. According to WebMD, "some early research suggests that using a Cannabidiol spray under the tongue might improve pain and muscle tightness, tiredness, bladder control, mobility, or well-being and quality of life in patients with MS."

According to WebMD, CBD Oil offers varying degrees of benefits in terms of addressing other medical conditions. Some of those medical conditions that research is being conducted to determine just how useful CBD is include: Bipolar disorder, Dystonia, Epilepsy, Huntington's disease, Insomnia, Parkinson's disease, Schizophrenia, Smoking Cessation, and Social Anxiety Disorder.

The current research that has been conducted thus far has not shown conclusive evidence that there is any effect on Bipolar disorder. However, while this information offers no direct conclusion, there is still promising research that will determine if there are any long term benefits.

Dystonia is medical condition that affects the muscles and results in severe muscle contractions that are involuntary. CBD is offering promising results while in the beginning stages of research. There is more research that must be conducted but it is definitely a promising treatment for this devastating disease.

Epilepsy is a disorder that a lot of research data concludes that taking CBD Oil can help to prevent seizures in many individuals. There is also data out there that conflicts these results. However, with the many patient reviews and testimonies that have been promoted on specific TV shows that do their research; I believe that there is definitely benefit in the use of CBD Oil in those individuals who suffer from seizures. Seizures can be so debilitating and thus anything that can offer some type of relief is a cause I would like to continue researching in order to provide conclusive evidence of these benefits.

Insomnia is a big problem in our society today. Because we live in such a fast paced and sometimes stressful world, it is hard to turn off the thought processes when it is time to wind down. Also in the news we have seen the detrimental effects of those sleep medications such as Ambien. There have been reports that individuals while taking Ambien have been driving, having car accidents, sleep eating and more. I don't know about you, but when I'm sleeping, I would like to stay sleeping in the comfort of my own home.

CBD Oil at high doses have shown significant promise in current research. WebMD indicates that if an individual who is suffering from Insomnia takes 160 mg of Cannabidiol prior to going to sleep it can improve overall sleep. Cannabidiol does not help you fall asleep, it actually works by keeping you asleep after you fall asleep. These benefits will help a lot of individuals who suffer from Insomnia.

Parkinson's disease is another medical condition that CBD is showing great promise in the beginning stages of research. Parkinson's disease is a debilitating disease and it is caused by the imbalance of Dopamine in the brain. There is too little Dopamine present in the brain and this results in a variety of symptoms. WebMD indicates that taking Cannabidiol can improve the psychotic symptoms associated with Parkinson's disease.

One breakthrough that is very encouraging is the benefits that Cannabidiol has on patients that suffer from Schizophrenia. Schizophrenia is a mental health condition in which there is too much Dopamine produced and this results in an imbalance in the Dopamine in the brain. The goal is to bring that Dopamine level back to an equilibrium. Research is showing significant benefits that may even equal current anti-psychotic standard of care treatment. While it has not been approved for treatment as the standard of care, there is definitely promise in the usage of Cannabidiol in the treatment of Schizophrenia. One research study that showed these benefits stated by WebMD, "that taking Cannabidiol 4 times daily for 4 weeks improves psychotic symptoms and might be as effective as the antipsychotic medication Amisulpride."

Smoking cessation is another point that the consumption of Cannabidiol may offer benefits. Because CBD Oil can be vaporized and smoked through an inhaler, some research concluded that inhaling CBD Oil would reduce the amount of cigarettes smoked in a weeks time by almost half.

Social Anxiety Disorders are another medical condition in which the benefits of CBD Oil have been indicated through research. The research conducted concluded that in order to effectively address and treat Social Anxiety Disorder, the CBD had to be ingested at high doses. Those doses were approximately 400-600 mg. However, there is still more research to conduct.

These are just some of the list of medical conditions and symptoms that have been associated with benefits from the addition of CBD Oil or just CBD. There are definitely promising results when you look at the overall research that has been conducted to date. There is also room for more research to be conducted, and more clinical trials to be conducted before we can conclude that there are benefits that conclusively affect these specific medical conditions.

However, after reviewing the information provided I can definitely infer that there is promising results. CBD Oil can provide symptom relief and management of many medical conditions. We are looking to the future for alternative therapies that will offer safer and more effective results than traditional medicine has been to offer over decades. CBD Oil is offering promising benefits that can make a major difference in the lives of those who suffer from these symptoms and diseases

Medical Journals that offer research suggesting CBD's benefits

The gold standard in all medical research are the double-blinded, randomized, controlled clinical trials. When we have those developed trials, it is quite certain that there is irrefutable evidence that this specific drug or therapy has offered the desired results at a specific period of time. Right now, in the medical world we have not yet reached that level of certainty when it comes to CBD, but we are right in the process of creating these evidence-based trials that will prove the benefits of CBD.

One trial titled, "Cannabidiol: Pharmacology and potential therapeutic role in epilepsy and other neuropsychiatric disorders" written by Orrin Devinsky et. al., provides scientific information regarding the relationship of Cannabidiol to the treatment or management of those patients who present with Epilepsy and other neuropsychiatric diseases.

The study describes the results that were found after performing this trial. The results found that the non-psychoactive component of cannabis which is Cannabidiol, showed promising results in managing seizures in animal trials in the acute stages. Because this relationship between Cannabidiol and Epilepsy is rather recent, in medical terms, there is yet to be studies that have followed these animals for a chronic period of time. Therefore, we are unaware at this time of the benefits that Cannabidiol offers in management of Epilepsy over the long term. More research is needed in order to offer more conclusive results.

CBD was also found to offer benefits to those individuals suffering from neurodegenerative diseases. CBD has also been linked to anti-inflammatory benefits as well.

While CBD alone does show promise in managing epilepsy, it is thought when combined with the THC components, that there is a greater result in managing Epilepsy both short and long term. The overall take away from this particular study was that while there is definitely a relationship between Cannabidiol and the management of Epilepsy, there is still more research that must be completed in order to understand that relationship and to determine the long term benefits that may or may not be present.

Another article published in Medscape Internal Medicine, which is a very respected website in which many healthcare professionals use, is titled, "Medical Cannabis: Pharmacy Focus on Treatment Options for Neurologic Conditions" written by Deborah Berblekamp. The journal article published in US Pharmacist Journal addresses the relationship between medical marijuana, which includes both THC and Cannabidiol, and various diseases in which traditional therapies have failed. Over the past several years there has been an increase in research looking at the benefits associated with alternative therapies.

First, as we have discussed medical marijuana contains many contents, but two of the components that offer the most medical benefits are: THC and Cannabidiol. THC is the psychoactive portion of the cannabis plant, and results in the "recreational high" that people misuse for that specific reason. The other component is Cannabidiol which is the non-psychoactive portion of the cannabis plant and can be extracted from many different areas of the cannabis plant. Cannabidiol is the component that will not result in any "high."

As we look at this journal article, we understand that there is constant research being done in order to prove that for these diseases that have failed traditional therapies, we need a new standard of care. This new standard of care that will offer these patients who have consistently and constantly suffered, to have hope that a new treatment has been researched and proven to offer benefits that other traditional therapies have not offered in the past.

Some of those diseases and disorders that CBD has been proven to offer promising benefits include: seizures, pain, muscle spasms, offer neuro-protection against neurodegenerative diseases, and has even been proven to reduce neuronal damage. Other diseases in which this medical therapy has been associated with either managing or decreasing the symptoms include the following: Parkinson's disease and ALS (Amyotrophic Lateral Sclerosis).

Do you understand how medically promising these findings are, and the opportunities for medical advancement we now have? Parkinson's disease and ALS (Amyotrophic Lateral Sclerosis) are diseases that decrease the quality of life for those that suffer with them. ALS has been in the news a lot lately because of the fundraisers that have been taking place. The "Ice Bucket Challenge" was a challenge to poor ice cold water on your head, and in doing so would raise money for this debilitating disease.

ALS is a progressive disease that affects the motor neurons of the central nervous system. These motor neurons are what allows us to move our muscles without even thinking. ALS also known as Lou Gehrig's disease is terminal and individuals who have this disease become progressively paralyzed.

Through this research conducted, there has been promising results that medical marijuana including the components THC and Cannabidiol offers neuron protection, and even reduce neuronal damage. While, it is not a cure for the disease, if through this treatment the reduction of damage to the motor neurons can be halted or slowed down, then this would increase the lifespans of those who suffer from this disease. We have to remember that this is just preliminary research, and results will vary. However, the research is very promising and we can look to this treatment as an opportunity to help those with this disease, and provide hope to those who are suffering from ALS.

Dr. Berlekamp, whom is a Pharmacist, in her journal article, continues to address that there are still federal restrictions on the use of medical cannabis; however, many states are suggesting specific recommendations concerning the medical use of cannabis.

One similarity that has been noticed across the variety of medical and scientific research conducted, is that the benefits associated with CBD and CBD Oil is basically dependent on the dosage and frequency taken. Therefore, it is imperative that a personalized treatment plan is developed based on the medical conditions or symptoms that are present in order to determine the dosage that will provide the most benefits. The dosing and frequency varies; and is determined based on a multitude of factors. Let's take a look and determine the appropriate doses of CBD for treatment purposes.

Dosing and Frequency of CBD?

As with any new medication healthcare professionals have to learn along with the other individuals involved in either the development of the medication, or in how to prescribe it once it has been approved for therapeutic treatment. Because CBD Oil is new, as far as being used in a controlled environment and prescribed by healthcare providers, there is a lot to learn about the dosing and frequency in which this medication should be recommended.

WebMD is a reputable website that discusses the dosage of Cannabidiol Oil, and it is stated that it is probably safe. WebMD stands behind this statement as long as the following recommendations are followed: CBD taken by mouth or sublingual through a spray. The specific dosage identified by WebMD to be a safe dose to take orally by mouth is up to 300 mg per day for a time period of no more than 6 months. Doses between 1200-1500 mg taken by mouth per day short term no longer than 4 weeks time period. For the CBD sublingual, or under the tongue, doses include 2.5 mg daily for a time period of 2 weeks.

These are recommendations, and individuals vary when taking medications or supplements that have not been scientifically researched to the fullest degree. Therefore, a dose that may be recommended, or even a smaller dose could have potentially higher effects on a patient not used to this component.

One such recommendation site titled, CBDOILREVIEW.ORG states that

they recommend a beginning standard dosage of 25 mg of CBD to be taken twice a day. Titration is key in order to determine the appropriate dosage that will provide the most benefits for the specific medical conditions.

CBD Oil offers recommended dosages based on the type of medical condition that you wish to treat. CBDOILREVIEW.ORG recommends the following dosages for the following medical conditions. Let's discuss a few of these conditions in depth.

If you or someone you know have had cancer in the past, or are currently facing this horrific diagnosis, it is quite a generalized understanding that appetite is the last thing on your mind. Many individuals who are suffering from cancer, whether it is breast cancer or lymphoma, a person's appetite is diminished. When cancer has reared its ugly head, it is imperative that calorie intake is actually increased and this can be difficult for individuals who do not have an appetite. Also, traditional treatment therapies including chemotherapy and radiation therapy can have synergistic effects on one's appetite as well; making it almost non-existent.

Thus, healthcare providers are constantly looking for a way to increase a individual who is suffering from cancer's appetite. Whether it is through medication or insertion of a gastric tube, it is imperative that cancer patients receive the proper nutrition. One recommended alternative therapy to some of the invasive treatments include the consumption of CBD Oil. Through many research studies, it has been proven that CBD Oil at a specific dosage has offered the benefit of increasing an individual's appetite. The dosage recommendation by CBDOILREVIEW.ORG is 2.5 mg of THC by mouth with 1 mg of CBD for 6 weeks. This is just one study that has provided a recommended dosage.

However, there are research studies being conducted almost daily that provide specific dosing regimens. Therefore, be sure to speak with a healthcare provider or Pharmacist in order to determine the most up to date recommendations for this medication.

Chronic pain is another disorder that has been increasing across our nation the past several years. Many individuals suffer from this debilitating disease on a daily basis, and are seeking alternative therapies because the traditional therapies are not offering any benefit. Most individuals who are suffering from chronic pain are on specific medication regimens and receiving epidural injections, or a variety of other types of injections just to try and maintain one day of relief. However, these invasive procedures in some cases do not offer the patient any pain relief, and in a lot of instances the patient has more pain after the procedure.

I have heard many patient's testimonies and they have specifically said that they wished there was something not invasive that would offer benefits without all the side effects and toxins associated with either medication or injection therapies. These patients suffering from painful diseases and disorders have one thing in common and that they just want to feel better. They just want to have one day in which they don't experience the debilitating and life altering pain. Well, through research and constant breakthroughs CBD has now been recommended to treat chronic pain. According to CBDOILREVIEW.ORG chronic pain can be treated with a starting dose of 2.5 mg of CBD daily for approximately 25 days.

The recommended dosage according to CBDOILREVIEW.ORG can be increased to 20 mg of CBD once daily. Once again, treatment recommendations can vary based on the new research that is constantly evolving, so be sure to check with the appropriate healthcare professionals in order to determine if this is still a therapeutic dosage. Also, because there is such a gap in the range from 2.5 mg to 25 mg daily, an appropriate dosage should be developed based on the patient's treatment plan.

We have discussed the importance of CBD Oil treatment in patients who suffer from epileptic seizures. The CBDOILREVIEW.ORG recommends that to treat epilepsy a high dosage of CBD Oil is required. The dosage range is between 200-300 mg to be taken by mouth once daily for up to 4 months. There have been many studies conducted that have linked the benefits of CBD Oil to the treatment and management of symptoms associated with epilepsy.

Therefore, it is a great opportunity for patients who suffer from this debilitating and life altering disease to benefit from this recommended dosage. Traditional pharmacologic therapies associated with the treatment of epilepsy have significant side effects and can in some cases even be toxic. Therefore, to find an alternative therapy that in the research conducted so far, seems to be a safe therapy, is a great benefit.

Huntington's disease is a that is terminal and destroys the nerve cells in the brain. It is a progressive and debilitating disease that results in death. It is a genetic disease and has no cure. Therefore, being diagnosed with this disease can have a serious impact both physically and psychologically on those individuals. Therefore, the being able to tell those patients who suffer from this disease that this new medical breakthrough may result in slowing down this debilitating process, and in some cases can even offer neuroprotection is an amazing message to deliver. As we understand there is no cure; but any alternative therapy that may offer benefits is worth a try.

The recommended dosage from CBDOILREVIEW.ORG states the treatment for Huntington's disease is 10 mg per kilogram of weight of CBD by month, once daily for 6 weeks. The recommendation provided, is just that, it is a recommendation and actual results will vary. This medication is still in research and so these results have not been conclusively understood. So, make sure that anytime you add any medication, whether it is a supplement or an over the counter medication, you need to speak with your healthcare provider to make sure there are not any interactions or other reasons why you should not implement this therapy into your treatment regimen.

Multiple Sclerosis is another central nervous disease that could potentially benefit from both components of medical marijuana. The CBDOILREVIEW.ORG recommends the treatment for Multiple Sclerosis should be between 2.5-120 mg of THC-CBD taken by mouth, once daily for 2 to 15 weeks. Other recommendations besides taking this as an oral medication, is to use the mouth spray as the route for this medication. CBDOILREVIEW.ORG recommends a spray that contains 2.7 mg of THC/2.5 mg of CBD for dosage of 2.5-120 mg for up to 8 weeks. The directions given by this website indicate that with the above formation of THC-CBD mouth spray, the patient can spray the contents up to 8 times in a 3 hour period of time.

The maximum amount of sprays that can be administered within a 24 hour period is 48 sprays. As you can see there are alternative therapies that are providing beneficial results in management of symptoms associated with Multiple Sclerosis. MS is a central nervous system disorder in which the nerves of the brain and spinal cord are being destroyed. Each nerve has a protective covering that allows for the fast transmittance of information across that covering. When this covering is disrupted or destroyed, the signals cannot be transmitted across any longer, and the result is the inability to move certain muscles. It is a progressive disease that interferes with the ability of a individual to move, when it has progressed.

It is a debilitating disease, and so any alternative therapy that would offer any benefits to this disease is a great alternative therapy to look into. As we have said prior, that this information is in the beginning stages of research, and there have not been any double-blinded, randomized, controlled trials that have been conducted yet. Therefore, we must understand results will vary. However, the research is very promising and if we continue to conduct this research and receive the information shown now, then this will be a medical breakthrough that so many individuals have been looking and hoping to find.

There are many more diseases and symptoms that CBD is offering beneficial results. Some of those include treating insomnia, schizophrenia, and glaucoma. Many individuals suffer from insomnia and are even on medications to make them sleep at night. Others who prefer to stay away from any prescription sleep medication, have tried hormones such as Melatonin to help them remain asleep. However, in both cases unwanted side effects or ineffectiveness of products has occurred thus resulting in unsatisfied and sleepy individuals.

The recommendation given by CBDOILREVIEW.ORG has found that if between 40-160 mg of CBD orally, once daily it will treat insomnia or other sleep disorders. Schizophrenia is another mental health disorder that many individuals suffer from. This disorder is an imbalance in Dopamine within the brain. It is recommended by CBDOILREVIEW.ORG that between 40-1,280 mg of CBD given orally, once daily for up to 4 weeks should offer some benefit in treating this disorder. Finally, Glaucoma is disorder that can result in many detrimental health conditions associated with an individual's eyes.

There are also different types of glaucoma, and because there is not a any distinguishing information given based on the treatment, it is imperative you speak with your physician concerning the appropriate dosage. It is also imperative to remember that Acute Angle Glaucoma is a medical emergency, and it is imperative you seek immediate medical attention to make sure that as a patient you protect your eyes; because a consequence of Acute Angle Glaucoma can be blindness. The dosage given by CBDOILREVIEW.ORG states that in order to treat glaucoma, a dose of between 20-40 mg, taken sublingually (under the tongue), one time only. There has been some research conducted that indicates higher dosages above the 40 mg dose, can actually precipitate increased eye pressures.

As with all medications, when beginning something new, it is imperative to continue to perform your research. Speak with your healthcare provider to determine the appropriate dosage for your unique medical treatment plan. No two individuals are the same and so we must remember that when doing this research. All of this information provided based on dosing is in the beginning stages of research, and have not been approved by the FDA; therefore, it is imperative that we speak with our healthcare providers to determine the appropriate dose for our specific medical treatment plan.

After reviewing this information both through the CBDOILREVIEW.ORG and through the information provided on MayoClinic the doses are provided based on the clinical research and clinical trials that have been conducted thus far. One disclaimer that MayoClinic places on their website is the same as we have been stating in this paper, "doses are based on scientific research, publications, traditional use, or expert opinion. Many herbs and supplements have not been thoroughly tested, and safety and effectiveness may not be proven. Brands may be made differently, with variable ingredients, even within the same brand."

It is imperative to be educated on the medications or supplements you are taking. The reviews and and research are pointing in the direction that Cannabidiol is a component of the Cannabis plant that offers great benefits for individuals who suffer from diseases that are debilitating and even life-threatening in many cases. The use of CBD for treatment of medical conditions is a scientific breakthrough.

How does it compare to Keppra in safety and side effects?

Keppra is a name brand medication classified as a anticonvulsant used in the treatment of seizures. Medscape is a reference that is used to determine nationally recommended doses of medications for specific medical conditions. Keppra, its generic name is Levetiracetam, it is used to treat a variety of different seizures. Keppra has been approved to treat adults who have Myoclonic Seizures. The recommended dosage is 500 mg by mouth, taken twice daily; every 12 hours. Dosage may be titrated to a therapeutic amount over time. This medication is also used in addition to other medications to treat partial onset seizures. Keppra can be used in adults to treat primary generalized tonic clonic seizures.

Pediatric treatments using Keppra for treatments of seizures is based on age and weight. Treatment of Myoclonic Seizures has not been studied and established in children less than 12 years of age. Children greater than 12 years of age, the treatment recommendation is 500 mg by mouth every 12 hours; and titrate by increasing 500 mg every 12 hours every 2 weeks to a recommended dose of 1500 mg every 12 hours. Keppra can be used to treat Primary Generalized Tonic-Clonic Seizures for ages 6 years and over. In treatment of partial onset seizures Keppra safety has not been established in infants less than 1 month. However, Keppra can be used in pediatric patients greater than 1 month of age for partial onset seizures; and the specific dosing is based on the infants weight and age; and must be titrated to a therapeutic level.

Keppra is not approved for some pediatric patients and so it is imperative to speak with a healthcare provider before incorporating this medication into one's healthcare treatment regiment. There are several interactions that range from severe to minor. As described by Medscape, there are 21 medications that have minor interactions with Keppra. There are three drugs that must be monitored closely because of their significant interactions that can occur. There are many known side effects associated with the medication Keppra. Some of those adverse reactions that are present in greater than 10% of those individuals who are taking this medication include: headache, infection, elevated blood pressure, fatigue, drowsiness, anorexia, weakness, cough, and weakness. There are many adverse reactions ranging from minor to serious and even life-threatening.

Keppra has been FDA approved, and is a therapy that has been treating seizures for years. There has been several studies that have proven its effectiveness. With that time, there has also been time for the various side effects and adverse reactions to be identified. Because of the amount of research that has been conducted when Keppra was developed, we have an understanding of the short term and long term side effects that may be present.

In comparison to CBD Oil, because it has not been researched for a extended period of time, we are unable to determine the long term effects or benefits of this component. Therefore, we are only able to acknowledge what we know at this point in the research process.

What we know so far is that there are minimal side effects when taken at the designated doses. We also know that there seems to be great benefits for a variety of diseases which includes seizures. Right now if we were to compare the information we have between Keppra and CBD Oil we can say that CBD Oil offers less side effects and less adverse reactions than Keppra. We, however, cannot comment on the long term, extended side effects and adverse reactions at this time, because we do not have the research to back it up.

Conclusion

CBD Oil is offering great promise in the research world. There is going to be constantly some form of controversy surrounding the various components of the cannabis plant for many more years to come. However, we are beginning to see that there is more to the cannabis plant then just THC. Now, we have established that Cannabidiol is another component of the cannabis plant that has great potential for medical and therapeutic uses.

We must continue to perform our due diligence and require the gold standard research and create double-blinded, randomized, controlled clinical trials. Once we have these established trials determining without a doubt the effects that we know CBD already offers, we can really begin to make a difference in the medical world.

CBD through the research that has already been conducted, we have found that it offers many benefits to those suffering from a wide variety of diseases. Some of those diseases include: chronic pain, chronic fatigue syndrome, Multiple Sclerosis, Huntington's disease, Parkinson's disease, ALS (Amyotrophic Lateral Sclerosis), and many others.

A lot of those diseases are terminal diseases in which there is no current cure. Individuals with those diseases have tried every type of therapy out there, and they have all failed to provide efficient benefits. CBD has shown to offer significant benefits to those individuals who suffer from these diseases on a daily basis. If this product can offer benefits and even management of symptoms to these individuals who suffer from these horrific diseases, then we can be witnesses of a huge medical breakthrough. Cannabidiol is a component of the cannabis plant, and it has the potential to make a huge difference in the lives of others.

Thank you for purchasing "CBD Hemp Oil" we would like to offer you a free gift!! Visit http://www.earthlymist.com/products/ and enter AZCBD to receive 20% off your first purchase of CBD Hemp Oil.

Information is gathered from the following sources:

https://healthyhempoil.com/cannabidiol-legal-status/

http://www.webmd.com/vitamins-supplements/ingredientmono-1439-cannabidiol.aspx?activeingredientid=1439&activeingredientname=cannabidiol

https://healthyhempoil.com/cannabidiol-side-effects/

http://www.leafscience.com/2014/02/23/5-must-know-facts-cannabidiol-cbd/

http://emedicine.medscape.com/article/1146199-overview

http://www.webmd.com/vitamins-supplements/ingredientmono-1439-cannabidiol.aspx?activeingredientid=1439&activeingredientname=cannabidiol

http://www.ncbi.nlm.nih.gov/pmc/articles/PMC4707667/

http://www.medscape.com/viewarticle/860049

http://www.mayoclinic.org/drugs-supplements/marijuana/dosing/hrb-20059701

https://cbdoilreview.org/cbd-cannabidiol/cbd-dosage/

http://www.clevelandclinicmeded.com/medicalpubs/diseasemanageme nt/neurology/epileptic-syndrome/

http://reference.medscape.com/drug/keppra-spritam-levetiracetam-343013#0

http://www.cannabis.info/gb/abc/10006556-how-to-make-cbd-oil&hloc=1

www.ingramcontent.com/pod-product-compliance
Lightning Source LLC
Chambersburg PA
CBHW072140290526
45789CB00013B/1648